WITHDRAWN

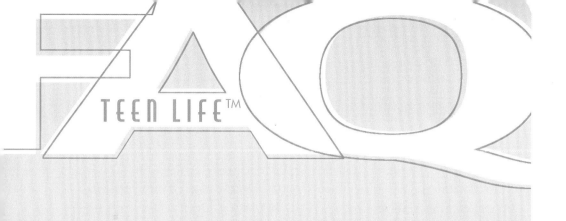

TEEN LIFE™

FREQUENTLY ASKED QUESTIONS ABOUT

Skin Cancer

John M. Shea, M.D.

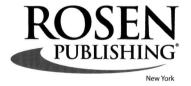

ROSEN
PUBLISHING®
New York

For my father, who has shown that having cancer should never stop one from living life to its fullest

Published in 2013 by The Rosen Publishing Group, Inc.
29 East 21st Street, New York, NY 10010

Library of Congress Cataloging-in-Publication Data

Shea, John M.
Frequently asked questions about skin cancer/John M. Shea.—1st ed.
    p. cm.—(FAQ: teen life)
Includes bibliographical references and index.
ISBN 978-1-4488-8327-1 (library binding)
1. Skin—Cancer—Popular works. 2. Skin—Cancer—Miscellanea. I. Title.
RC280.S5S53 2013
616.99'477—dc23

2012014436

Manufactured in the United States of America

CPSIA Compliance Information: Batch #W13YA: For further information, contact Rosen Publishing, New York, New York, at 1-800-237-9932.

WHAT IS SKIN CANCER?

Human skin is truly amazing. As the largest organ, skin covers the body from head to toe. It provides the first line of defense against disease-causing bacteria, toxic chemicals, and extreme temperatures of the outside environment. Nerve endings in the skin allow us to learn about the world around us through our sense of touch. Waterproof skin keeps fluids inside the body. Skin cells have a very active metabolism: new skin cells are constantly being made, while old, dead cells are shed off. Skin cells also produce vitamin D, a nutrient that is vital for strong bones and teeth.

Unfortunately, the skin is at risk for developing cancer, a disease in which a group of cells grows uncontrollably. Growth is necessary for every cell. Under normal circumstances, cells grow in a tightly controlled manner. Chemical signals tell healthy cells when to stop growing.

Just as brakes are important for the safety of a car, the signals for cells to stop growing are important for the health of an organ system. Cancerous cells no longer respond to these signals to stop, and therefore they grow out of control.

This group of abnormal cells may become large enough to form a mass, or tumor, which can disrupt the function of healthy cells nearby. Sometimes, cancer cells can metastasize, or spread, and begin growing in other organs. There are many different types of skin cancers (sometimes referred to as skin carcinomas), depending on the type of skin cells from which the cancer first grows. Each type of cancer behaves in a unique way and has a different prognosis (expected outcome or prospect for recovery).

Understanding the anatomy of human skin will help us better understand the different types of skin cancer. It is important to keep in mind that these classifications help us understand how a disease is expected to behave, but not always how it will behave. Each case of cancer is as unique as the person affected by it.

The Anatomy of Skin

Skin is made up of three distinct layers: epidermis, dermis, and subcutaneous tissue. The outermost layer, the epidermis, is about as thick as a sheet of paper. This is the layer that is most exposed to the harsh environments outside the body. The most abundant cells in the epidermis are known as keratinocytes (the suffix "-cyte" means "cell"). These cells make a protein called keratin that helps strengthen and protect the skin. Keratin is also a chief component

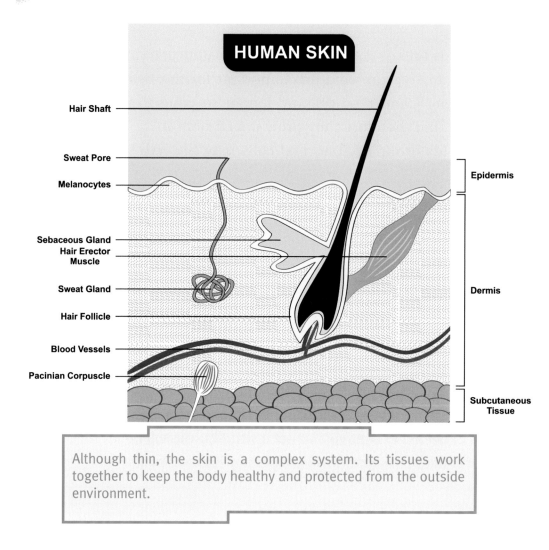

HUMAN SKIN

Hair Shaft

Sweat Pore

Melanocytes

Sebaceous Gland
Hair Erector
Muscle

Sweat Gland

Hair Follicle

Blood Vessels

Pacinian Corpuscle

Epidermis

Dermis

Subcutaneous
Tissue

Although thin, the skin is a complex system. Its tissues work together to keep the body healthy and protected from the outside environment.

of fingernails and hair. Another important protein in this layer is melanin, a dark pigment that gives skin its color. Melanin protects skin cells by absorbing dangerous ultraviolet (UV) radiation from sunlight. When skin is exposed to high levels of UV radiation, cells called melanocytes produce more melanin to absorb more UV radiation, making skin tan.

The next layer, the dermis, is much thicker than the epidermis. In addition to skin cells, the dermis contains hair follicles, sweat glands, nerve endings, and blood vessels. The dermis contains two important proteins: elastin and collagen. Elastin gives skin its flexibility. It is the reason why skin returns to its normal form after it is pinched or pulled. Collagen gives skin its shape and strength. Collagen and elastin tend to break down over time, making the skin sag as people age.

The deepest skin layer is the subcutaneous tissue (sometimes referred to as the hypodermis). This layer is chiefly composed of collagen, fibroblasts (cells that make collagen), and fat cells. The collagen functions to strengthen the skin, while fat cells provide insulation by trapping heat inside the body. In addition, the fat layer acts as a cushion, protecting the inner organs from injuries.

Melanoma

Most skin cancers are classified into two major categories: melanomas and keratinocytic cancers. Melanomas are tumors that arise from melanocytes. These tumors usually appear dark brown or black, although sometimes they may appear flesh-colored or even white. Often, they appear in sun-exposed areas of the body, especially the neck and face, but they can also appear on the soles of the feet, on the palms of the hands, under nail beds, and even in parts of the eye. Among men, melanomas usually appear on the chest or back, while among women they often are found on the legs.

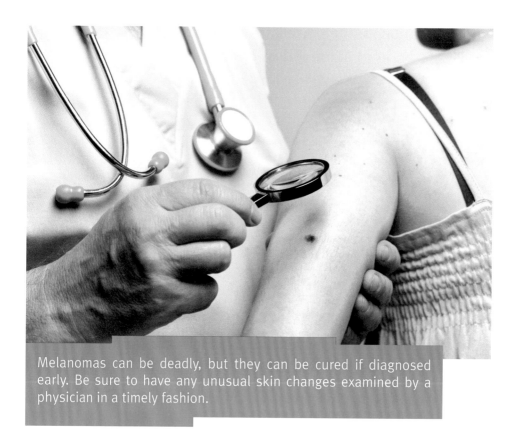

Melanomas can be deadly, but they can be cured if diagnosed early. Be sure to have any unusual skin changes examined by a physician in a timely fashion.

Melanomas may resemble a simple mole, which is a benign, or harmless, concentration of melanocytes in a small area of skin. Unfortunately, unlike moles, melanomas are malignant, meaning that the tumor will continue to grow and spread if not treated. Melanomas may even spread to internal organs. They are the most dangerous form of skin cancer and carry the poorest prognosis if they are unrecognized and untreated.

People who have large or numerous moles on their body are at a higher risk of developing melanomas. It is always prudent to watch moles for worrisome changes. The American Academy of

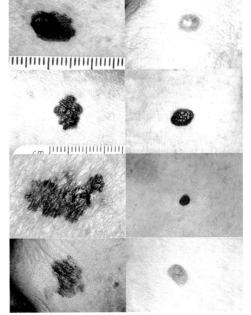

Dermatology recommends the ABCDE approach to evaluating a suspicious mole:

- **A**symmetry. Is each half of the mole the mirror image of the other?
- **B**order. Is the border of the mole smooth?
- **C**olor. Is the mole the same color throughout?
- **D**iameter. Is the diameter smaller than a pencil eraser?
- **E**volving. Does the mole look the same each time it is examined?

Answering "no" to any of these questions should prompt an immediate evaluation by a health care provider.

According to the American Cancer Society (ACS), more than seventy thousand Americans are diagnosed with melanomas every year. While melanomas account for less than 5 percent of all skin cancers, they can be deadly, especially if they are ignored as benign moles. About 75 percent of all skin cancer–related deaths are caused by melanomas, according to the ACS.

According to projections from the National Cancer Institute (NCI), approximately 8,790 Americans were expected to die from melanoma in 2011; that is about one death every hour. In 2012, more than nine thousand people were expected to die from the disease. On the other hand, many melanomas that are recognized and treated early can be cured completely.

According to the ACS, rates of melanoma have been increasing over the past thirty years. In addition, the American Melanoma Foundation (AMF) reports that melanoma is the second most common form of cancer for teens and young adults ages fifteen to twenty-nine. According to the NCI, about seven out of every one thousand melanoma diagnoses are made in people under age twenty. An article in the *Journal of Clinical Oncology* reports that rates of melanoma among children and teens, especially teenage girls, are increasing every year.

Keratinocytic Carcinoma

Most skin cancers initially come from abnormal keratinocytes. Because the presentation, aggressiveness, prognosis, and treatment of these cancers are very different from melanomas, they are sometimes referred to as non-melanoma skin cancers.

Keratinocytic carcinomas are by far the most common type of cancer. According to the ACS, about 2.2 million new cases of non-melanoma skin cancers are diagnosed every year. Luckily, non-melanomas are much less deadly than melanomas. Keratinocyte carcinomas are responsible for about two thousand deaths a year. The two types of keratinocyte cancers are basal cell carcinoma and squamous cell carcinoma.

According to the American Medical Association (AMA), basal cell carcinoma (BCC) accounts for about three-quarters of all skin cancers. Indeed, it is the most common of all cancers among humans. The abnormal keratinocytes come from the lowest layer of cells in the epidermis, known as the basal cell layer. The tumors are typically found on sun-exposed areas of the face and neck. They often appear as waxy red bumps with a depression on top, like a volcano (though other presentations can occur).

Traditionally, BCCs are associated with older adults, not children and youth. But increasingly, younger people are being diagnosed with this cancer, perhaps due to the increased popularity of tanning. Because BCC is typically a slow-growing cancer and rarely metastasizes, the mortality rate is low. Left untreated, BCCs can grow and invade nearby organs, such as muscles and bones. Even with successful treatment, BCC has a high rate of recurrence. According to the ACS, about one-half of people with BCC will develop a new skin cancer within five years.

After BCC, the second most common type of skin cancer is squamous cell carcinoma (SCC), which accounts for about 20 percent of skin cancers, according to the American Society of Clinical Oncology (ASCO). SCC develops from abnormal keratinocytes in the upper layers of the epidermis. Compared to BCC, SCC grows more quickly and is much more likely to

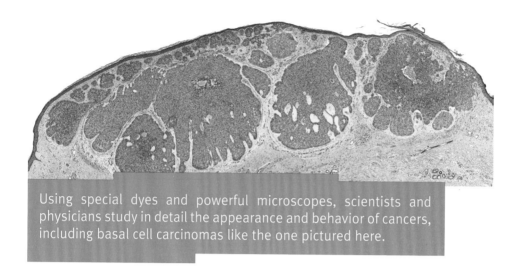

Using special dyes and powerful microscopes, scientists and physicians study in detail the appearance and behavior of cancers, including basal cell carcinomas like the one pictured here.

metastasize. However, the mortality rate is low if it is caught early. When a squamous cell tumor is still small and has not yet invaded the deeper dermis, it is known as squamous cell carcinoma in situ, or Bowen's disease.

SCC can typically be found in sun-exposed areas of the skin, including the face, lips, neck, and ears. The tumor often appears flat with crusting skin (though, like other skin cancers, presentation can vary). Exposure to some chemicals can cause SCC to appear in other places, such as on the hands or, in the case of cigarette smokers, inside the mouth.

Actinic keratoses are small, rough patches of skin found in areas of sun exposure, including the face, ears, hands, and scalp. They are more common among the elderly, especially those with lighter skin and a history of multiple sunburns. Actinic keratoses are often benign. However, according to the University of Maryland Medical Center, in 5 percent of cases they may develop into SCC, and thus they may be considered precancerous. Treatments for actinic keratoses are simple, and a physician often removes them from the body during the same visit as the diagnosis. Actinic keratoses that are not removed are routinely checked for worrisome changes.

Uncommon Skin Cancers

Melanomas, BCCs, and SCCs together account for more than 99 percent of all skin cancers, according to the ACS. A much more rare form of skin cancer is Merkel cell carcinoma. This cancer grows from hormone-producing cells found in the skin.

According to the Seattle Cancer Care Alliance, recent studies suggest that these cells may become cancerous because of a virus called Merkel cell polyomavirus (MCV). Interestingly, MCV is a common virus, and many people are infected with it with very few symptoms. For reasons not well understood, however, this virus may cause skin cells to become cancerous in a small number of people.

Merkel cell carcinoma typically occurs in people older than sixty-five and in people with compromised immune systems, such as those with HIV/AIDS, those with certain types of leukemia, or those who have taken medications that suppress immunity (as in the case of organ transplantation).

Kaposi's sarcoma is another uncommon cancer. It typically originates in the dermis, and it appears to be caused by human herpesvirus 8 (HHV-8). Several decades ago, it was a very rare cancer, mostly limited to the elderly and those of Mediterranean origin. Since the 1980s, however, it has become more common among people with weak immune systems, especially those with HIV/AIDS.

Lymphomas are cancers that start from immune cells called lymphocytes. Lymphocytes are found all over the body, especially inside bones and inside small, infection-fighting organs called lymph nodes. There are some lymphocytes in the skin, and when these become cancerous, it is known as primary cutaneous lymphoma. While lymphomas are typically more common among older adults, it is not uncommon for a child or young adult to develop this type of lymphoma.

WHAT CAUSES SKIN CANCER?

Cells in our bodies are constantly growing, dividing, resting, and dying. Cell death is critical for a healthy body. Worn-out and damaged cells must be removed to make room for younger, healthier cells. The cells in the epidermal layer of skin die and are replaced about every twenty-eight days. Millions of dead skin cells are shed from the body every day (this material makes up a large part of the dust in the air around us).

Cells receive signals from both inside themselves and from other tissues that trigger their growth, rest, or death. Cancers arise when cells no longer respond to these signals but continue to grow and make copies of themselves in an unregulated manner. The copies also fail to respond to signals to stop growing, and so the cancer continues to grow and spread.

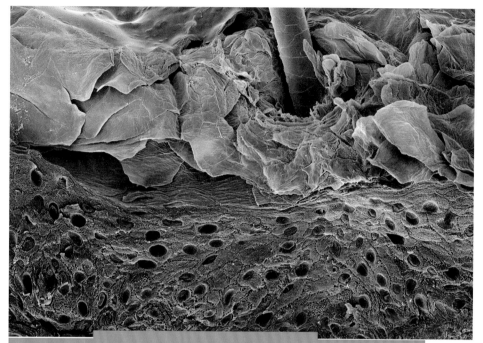

Scanning electron microscopes (SEMs) can show researchers greater detail than traditional light microscopes. In this SEM image, we see the outermost layer of flattened, dead skin cells surrounding a hair.

How a Cell Becomes Cancerous

The first step in turning a normal cell into a cancerous one begins with damage to its genetic blueprints: DNA. DNA contains information on when a cell should grow and divide, what type of cell to become, which proteins to make, and when to rest and die. This information can be corrupted in a number of ways. Sometimes, a mistake is made when a cell is copying its own DNA. This is known as a spontaneous mutation. In many cases, the damage is caused by something in the environment. High levels of radiation, including X-rays and UV radiation, have been shown to damage DNA and cause mutations. Chemicals such as tar, asbestos, and tobacco also corrupt genetic information. Research at the Mayo Clinic in Rochester, Minnesota, has shown that some viruses, such as the hepatitis B virus (HBV) and human papillomavirus (HPV), cause cancer by damaging DNA. When DNA becomes mutated, every copy that the dividing cell makes will also contain the mutation. If a mutation occurs in reproductive cells (sperm or eggs), there is a chance that one's children could also inherit the mutation in their own DNA.

The Genetics of Skin Cancer

Innovations in genetic research over the last half-century have allowed scientists to study in detail the causes of skin cancers. In SCC, for example, the most commonly mutated gene is known as the p53 gene. The p53 protein continually checks DNA for damage, and upon finding it, stops the cell from dividing and attempts to repair the DNA. If the DNA cannot be repaired, p53 signals the cell to self-destruct. Mutations in p53 that prevent this important function allow abnormal cells to continue to live and multiply.

In BCC, the most frequently affected gene is *PTCH* (pronounced "patched"). *PTCH* slows down the rate of growth and division in cells. When *PTCH* is damaged, cells are free to divide more quickly. Damage to *PTCH* can be acquired in some cells due to errors in DNA copying, UV radiation, or chemical damage to DNA. In a condition known as nevoid basal cell carcinoma syndrome (NBCCS), a person inherits a mutated *PTCH* gene from a parent, so every *PTCH* gene in that person's body is damaged. Those with NBCCS are more susceptible not only to skin cancers but to also cancers of other body organs, including the bones and organs of the central nervous system. NBCCS is a common cause of BCC among people under the age of twenty.

More than one-half of melanomas have a mutated *BRAF* gene. In normal cells, *BRAF* is part of a signaling network that tells a cell to grow and divide. When mutated, *BRAF* works too well, and the signal to multiply never gets turned off.

Other genes known to be connected to the risk of developing melanoma include *CDKN2A* and *CDK4*. Both work together to tightly control the rate at which a healthy cell divides. People with many close relatives who have had melanomas are often found to have inherited mutated *CDKN2A* or *CDK4* from their parents.

It is important to remember that mutations in DNA are cumulative, which means that small changes are passed from mother cells to daughter cells over years. New mutations can then occur in the already damaged cells, increasing the likelihood that a cell will become cancerous. Just as multiple misspellings in a sentence make it harder to understand its meaning, more mutations in a cell make it harder for the cell to behave normally. Scientists now understand that most cancerous cells contain several mutations in different genes that have accumulated over years. It is the combination of these mutations that results in uncontrolled cell growth and cancer.

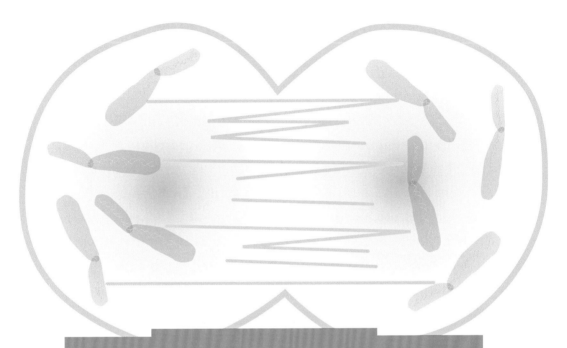

When cells divide, each daughter cell gets an exact copy of the mother cell's DNA. If the mother cell has a mutation, each daughter cell will inherit that mutation.

Carcinogens

There are billions of pieces of information encoded in human DNA, and cells do a remarkable job of copying this information faithfully. There are even proteins in cells whose job it is to "proofread" newly copied DNA and correct any mistakes they encounter. Even so, some mistakes are missed, and these changes are passed down each time the mutated cell divides.

Spontaneous mutations only account for a small percentage of mutations, however. There are many environmental substances or agents that have been shown to produce muta-tions and cause cancer. As the organ most exposed to the environment, the skin is particularly susceptible to a number of these carcinogens.

The chief cause of skin cell mutations is ultraviolet (UV) radi-ation. Although human eyes are not adapted to see UV radiation, it is a high-energy light. The most common sources of UV radiation are the sun and tanning beds. Two types of UV radiation are significant in the development of skin cancer: UVA, which has a longer wavelength and can penetrate skin deeply; and UVB, which has a shorter wavelength but higher energy. Although UVB cannot penetrate the skin as deeply, it is believed to be a greater cause of cancer than UVA.

Sunburns occur when UV radiation causes extensive dam-age to the DNA of epidermal cells, and these cells die in large numbers. There is a strong correlation between sunburns and skin cancer. However, it is important to remember that UV radiation can cause mutations in skin cells even without caus-ing sunburns.

Some people are more sensitive to the harmful effects of UV radiation than others. Xeroderma pigmentosum is a rare disease (about one in a million people have it) in which individuals can develop severe sunburns within minutes of sun exposure. It can take weeks for the skin to repair itself. For people with the dis-ease, sun exposure also causes dry skin (xeroderma) and changes in skin color (pigmentosum), including severe freck-ling. Many people with xeroderma pigmentosum will develop multiple skin cancers in their lifetime. About half will have their

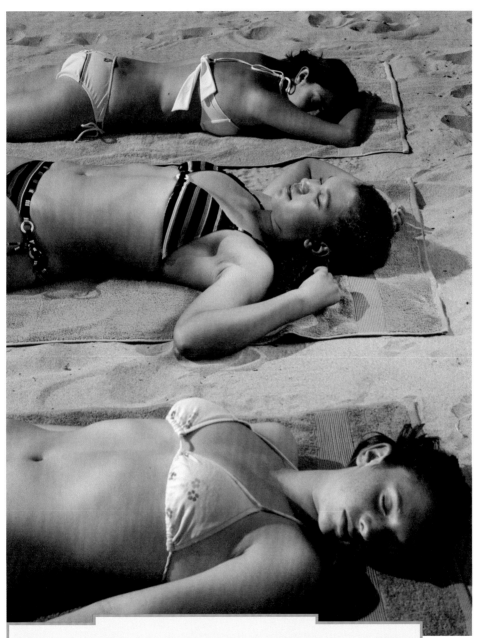

Rates of skin cancer are increasing among young women, most likely due to the popularity of tanning and increased UV radiation exposure.

first skin cancer by the age of ten. Xeroderma pigmentosum is a genetic disease inherited from both parents. In the case of this disease, proteins that repair UV-radiation-damaged DNA have been mutated. Thus, people are more susceptible to the cancer-causing effects of UV radiation.

There are a number of chemicals that have been linked to skin cancer. Coal, soot, tar, and pitch are all classified as polycyclic aromatic hydrocarbons (PAHs). PAHs have been linked to a number of cancers, including skin and lung cancers. Motor oil also contains PAHs, and repeated exposure to it has been shown to cause skin cancers in research animals. Arsenic is a naturally occurring chemical found in the environment, and some well water has been found to contain significant levels of this toxin. Pesticides and weed killers also contain significant levels of arsenic, as do some "all-natural" herbal remedies. Arsenic exposure has many deadly effects, including liver cancer and non-melanoma skin cancers.

Infection and Immunology

We have already learned that some viruses have been linked to skin cancers. According to an article in the *Journal of the National Cancer Institute*, scientists are hypothesizing a link between Merkel cell carcinoma and infection with the Merkel cell polyomavirus. Kaposi's sarcoma is caused by human herpesvirus 8.

According to *U.S. News & World Report*, there is growing evidence that human papillomavirus (HPV) raises the risk of developing squamous cell carcinoma. HPV is a very common virus, and many people are infected with it with few or no symptoms. In some people, HPV may produce the benign tumors commonly known as warts. Occasionally, however, HPV may trigger SCC development by interfering with proteins that signal cells to stop growing. Those with compromised immune systems, such as organ transplant recipients or those with AIDS, are especially susceptible.

The fact that the risks of cancer are much higher when the immune system is weakened illustrates just how important this system is in fighting cancer. The immune system can both recognize cancerous cells and kill them. While many immune cells and hormones contribute to this function, T cells and NK (natural killer) cells are among the most important. Healthy cells signal to T cells and NK cells that everything is working correctly inside. Cancerous cells, because of their damaged DNA and altered metabolism, frequently send abnormal signals to the immune cells. This triggers a response in the immune cells to kill the abnormal cells. These immune cells then release hormones that recruit other immune cells into the area to search for other cancer cells.

three

HOW CAN SKIN CANCER BE PREVENTED?

According to the American Academy of Dermatology, skin cancer diagnosis rates are increasing among adults under the age of forty, especially among young women. This is unfortunate, especially considering that scientists now have a better understanding of what causes skin cancer and how to prevent it. Lowering the chances of developing skin cancer begins with recognizing and minimizing the risk factors. There are several ways you can change your behavior to lower your risk.

One very important way to prevent skin cancer is to catch it while it is in a precancerous state. All types of skin cancers are highly curable if they are recognized and treated early enough. The ACS suggests that you "check your birthday suit on your birthday." This means that once a year, a person should examine the whole body for any skin changes or worrisome new growths. This includes moles that change in shape or color, or areas of the

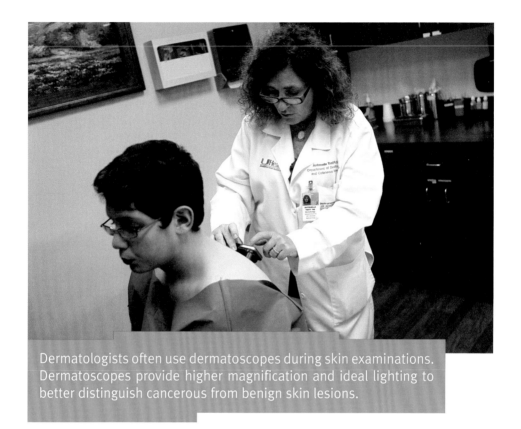

Dermatologists often use dermatoscopes during skin examinations. Dermatoscopes provide higher magnification and ideal lighting to better distinguish cancerous from benign skin lesions.

skin that are swelling, itching, or bleeding for unknown reasons. As part of normal health maintenance, your health care providers should do a similar whole-body examination yearly as well. People with many risk factors for skin cancer, or who have had skin cancer in the past, should perform these self-examinations more often.

What You Can't Change

Some risk factors for skin cancer cannot be modified. For example, having light skin is a risk factor for developing skin cancer. According to the ACS, white people are ten times more likely to get melanomas than African Americans. This makes sense when we consider that African American skin contains higher amounts of UV-radiation-blocking melanin than white skin does. People with light-colored eyes and people that freckle easily also appear to have a higher risk of skin cancer.

Likewise, having a close relative (such as a parent or a sibling) with skin cancer is also a risk factor that cannot be changed. There is a strong connection between family history and the development of melanomas. As mentioned previously, scientists have discovered mutated *CDKN2A* genes in families with higher incidences of melanomas. Scientists have also noted that people who inherit mutated *PTCH* genes tend to develop BCC very early in life. A number of other genes are suspected to play a role in the development of skin cancer and are currently being studied.

Chemical Exposure

We cannot change our skin color or our families, but there are risk factors for skin cancer that can be minimized. One of them is exposure to cancer-causing chemicals. Arsenic and PAHs are two chemicals that have been linked to an increased risk of various cancers, including skin cancers. The Occupational Safety and Health Administration (OSHA) requires industries, such as mining or smelting, that deal with these chemicals to provide protective equipment for their employees, including gloves, masks, and eyewear. In our homes, however, we must be responsible for our own health and safety. Motor oil and chimney soot are just two common sources of PAHs that many people may not realize are carcinogens. Therefore, they may not take the necessary precautions to protect themselves. Wearing gloves and long sleeves when dealing with such chemicals and thorough washing afterward are simple ways to help protect against chemical exposure.

Chemical exposure also occurs through tobacco use. A key by-product of cigarette and pipe smoke is tar, which is a PAH. According to the American Society of Clinical Oncology, smoking tobacco products more than triples one's risk for SCC. This risk increases the longer and more frequently someone smokes. Former smokers have almost twice the risk for developing SCC than people who have never smoked.

The High Risks of UV Radiation Exposure

Scientists universally agree that UV radiation exposure is the most important risk factor in the development of skin cancer. It is responsible for the vast majority of DNA damage that leads to cancer. Avoiding UV radiation is the simplest and most effective way to decrease one's chances of developing both melanomas and keratinocytic cancers.

The sun is the most important source of UV radiation in daily life. People must take care to avoid excessive exposure to the sun for long periods. Many people with skin cancer experienced multiple sunburns when they were young. In addition, scientists

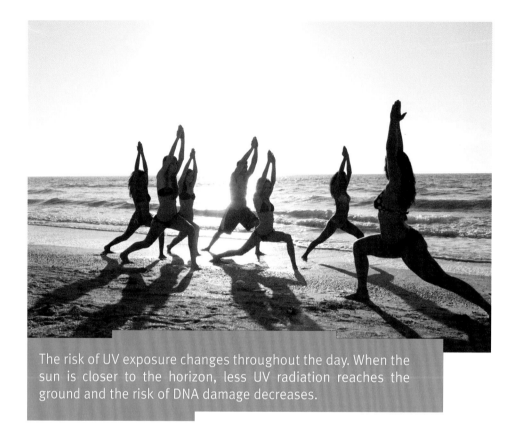

The risk of UV exposure changes throughout the day. When the sun is closer to the horizon, less UV radiation reaches the ground and the risk of DNA damage decreases.

now understand that even low levels of UV radiation exposure that does not result in sunburn can still damage DNA and lead to skin cancer.

UV radiation from the sun is strongest between the hours of 10 AM and 4 PM. The "shadow rule" is a good way to estimate the sun's intensity: if your shadow is shorter than you are, the sun's rays are at their most intense, and therefore the skin must be protected. You can remember this rule with the phrase, "Short shadow, seek shade!" This is true even on cloudy days—UV radiation may pass through the clouds even when visible sunlight is blocked.

The surface of the ground can influence how much of these damaging rays we are exposed to. Concrete, sand, and water are just some of the surfaces that reflect UV radiation back up to us. Freshly fallen snow is one of the worst offenders, reflecting nearly 85 percent of the radiation from the sun. That nearly doubles our UV radiation exposure and subjects us to UV radiation even when we are in the shade.

Location influences UV radiation exposure as well. The intensity of the solar radiation reaching Earth per square foot is greater when the sun is directly overhead than when it is closer to the horizon. Those living closest to the equator (where the sun is most directly overhead) receive the most UV radiation, while those closer to the northern or southern poles receive less. People who are born close to the equator (or who have ancestors from those areas) tend to have more UV-radiation-blocking melanin, and darker skin, as a result of the greater exposure.

People who live at higher altitudes also have higher UV radiation exposure. This is because there is a thinner atmosphere to absorb solar radiation, so more of it reaches the ground. According to Health Canada, at an elevation of 6,500 feet (1,981 meters), up to 30 percent more UV radiation reaches the ground than at sea level.

Avoiding excessive UV radiation means avoiding the sun's rays when they are most intense. Seek shade between the hours of 10 AM and 4 PM, and wear protective clothing. Good choices include long-sleeved shirts and hats with wide brims to cover and protect the neck and ears. Wear sunglasses that provide UV radiation protection. In addition to damaging skin, UV radiation can cause melanomas in the eye known as ocular melanomas.

Sunscreen and Sunblock

Sunscreen and sunblock offer significant protection against the damaging effects of UV radiation. Sunscreen is a specially formulated material (cream, lotion, or spray) that helps keep most UV radiation from reaching the skin. Some people use the term "sunscreen" interchangeably with suntan lotion or sunblock. Suntan lotion may refer to any material placed on the skin to prevent sunburns. These skin care products may or may not have any UV-radiation-blocking properties. In contrast, sunblock often has near-complete UV-radiation-blocking properties. Sunblock is most useful for people who burn easily and are at high risk for skin cancer.

The Food and Drug Administration (FDA) requires that a number called the sun protection factor (SPF) be included on sunscreen labels. This number indicates how well the product protects skin from the sun. Specifically, skin protected with an SPF 15 sunscreen takes fifteen times longer to redden or become sunburned than skin without sunscreen protection does. For example, if it takes 10 minutes for skin to turn red in the sun without sunscreen, it will take 2.5 hours (150 minutes) to turn red with an SPF 15 sunscreen. A product marked SPF 15 blocks about 93 percent of UVB rays, while a product marked SPF 30 blocks 97 percent of UVB rays.

Although some sunscreen manufacturers claim their products have an SPF of 60 or above, there is no evidence that these products provide any greater skin production than SPF 50. The FDA is proposing a new regulation that will cap the maximum

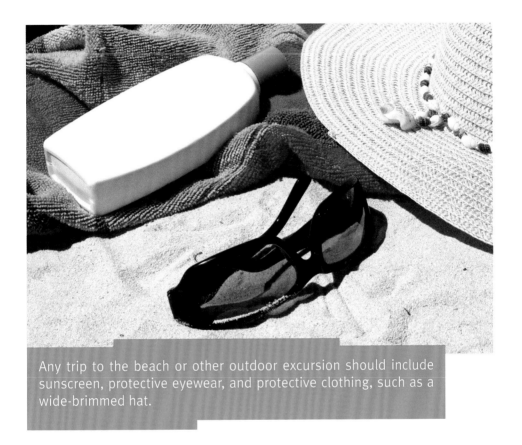

Any trip to the beach or other outdoor excursion should include sunscreen, protective eyewear, and protective clothing, such as a wide-brimmed hat.

SPF a manufacturer can claim on its labels at SPF 50+. In this way, consumers will not erroneously believe that a product marked SPF 75 will make them safer than one with SPF 50.

UVB rays are responsible for sunburns and for most of the DNA damage associated with skin cancer. However, UVA plays a smaller but significant role in DNA damage. The active ingredients in some older sunscreen (salicylates and cinnamates) do an excellent job blocking UVB but not UVA. Newer "broad-spectrum" sunscreen includes ingredients such as oxybenzone, titanium oxide, and zinc oxide that also block UVA radiation.

FDA regulations evaluate the strength of UVA protection with a four-star rating system. One star offers minimal UVA protection, while four stars offer the maximum UVA protection.

The Skin Cancer Foundation (SCF) recommends wearing SPF 15 daily for skin protection (or a higher SPF for those that burn easily or have a higher risk of skin cancer). The sunscreen should be applied thirty minutes before sun exposure to give the active ingredients time to bind to the skin. Water-resistant sunscreen is a great idea for the beach, pool, or very hot days when you may get sweaty, as it binds very well with the skin. On the other hand, water-resistant sunscreens may feel sticky and may interfere with makeup, so they may not be ideal for everyday use. FDA regulations now require sunscreen manufacturers to clearly label the amount of time a person may sweat or swim before a water-resistant sunscreen loses its SPF effectiveness. The label must specify either forty or eighty minutes of effectiveness, based on testing.

Sunscreen should be applied on all areas of exposed skin, including face, ears, and neck. A commonly neglected area is the top of the feet; this area is important to remember for those wearing flip-flops or sandals. Those with balding or shaved heads should protect the top of the head at all times. About 1 ounce (30 milliliters)—or about two tablespoons—of sunscreen should be applied to the whole body for those going to the beach. The SCF estimates that most people are only using half the recommended amount and are thus not getting full protection. In addition, the ingredients in sunscreen begin to lose effectiveness after about two hours. People should reapply sunscreen every other hour regardless of the instructions on the bottle.

All adults and all children over the age of six months should wear sunscreen daily no matter how long their sun exposure is. Children under the age of six months should avoid all sun exposure. They should wear protective clothing, including a wide-brim hat, and remain in the shade.

There are some, such as the Environmental Working Group (EWG), that claim commercially available sunscreen should be avoided as the ingredients may damage the skin. However, there is little evidence to support such claims, and indeed, plenty of scientific evidence confirms the safety of these products for humans. Others advocate "all-natural" alternatives to sunscreen, such as mango butter or shea butter, which contains cinnamate. While these products may have mild sun-blocking properties, they are not nearly as effective as FDA-regulated sunscreen and should not be considered a safe alternative.

The Risks of Tanning

The rate of skin cancer has been increasing, especially among young women. Scientists believe a large part of that trend is due to the growing popularity of tanning among teenagers and young adults. The AAD reports that four out of five young women frequently tan outdoors. The organization also reports that nearly a third of women visit a tanning booth yearly, and up to a quarter visit weekly. Many young people take vacations in sunny locations, further increasing their exposure to the harmful effects of the sun.

Some tanning salons claim that their tanning beds are a safe alternative to natural sun exposure. Some even promote

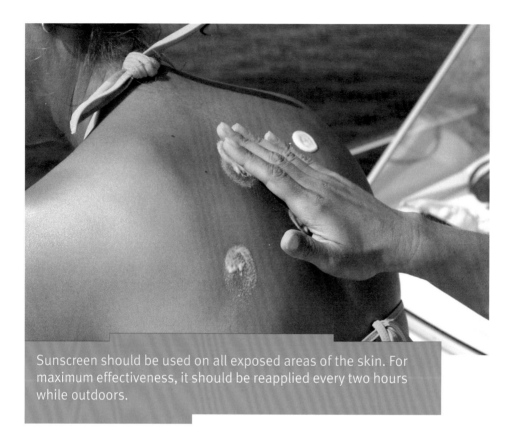

Sunscreen should be used on all exposed areas of the skin. For maximum effectiveness, it should be reapplied every two hours while outdoors.

indoor tanning as healthy, claiming it is a source of vitamin D. However, tanning beds produce UV radiation, which has DNA-damaging properties regardless of whether it comes from natural or artificial sources. Both the U.S. Department of Health and Human Services and the World Health Organization's International Agency of Research on Cancer have declared the UV radiation from tanning booths to be a known carcinogen. The American Academy of Pediatrics (AAP) is advocating laws to ban teenagers from using indoor tanning facilities.

Nutrition and Health

Nutrition has been proven to play a vital part in preventing skin cancer. Two of the most important nutrients identified have been vitamins C and E. Both are antioxidants, and both seem to minimize damage to DNA after UV radiation exposure. According to the *Journal of Investigative Dermatology*, a recent study showed that people who had been taking vitamins C and E had fewer sunburns and less evidence of DNA damage compared to those deficient in those vitamins. Of course, vitamin intake does not replace the use of sunscreen and UV-radiation-avoidance, but rather supplements them. These vitamins are protective against skin cancer and other effects of sun exposure, including premature aging and the appearance of wrinkles. Excellent sources of vitamin C include citrus fruit, broccoli, cauliflower, and leafy green vegetables. Vitamin E can be found in nuts, seeds, spinach, and asparagus. Because taking too much of these vitamins can be harmful, those who are considering taking vitamin supplements should talk to their health care provider first.

While it is not directly beneficial in protecting against skin cancer, vitamin A is important for the repair and maintenance of healthy skin. Vitamin A is found in dairy products, meat (especially liver), dark green leafy vegetables, and orange and yellow vegetables, such as carrots.

There is some controversy about sun exposure and vitamin D. The skin is able to make vitamin D when it is exposed to small amounts of UV radiation. Vitamin D is crucial for strong bones and teeth. It is also important for a healthy immune system, which is important in fighting cancers, including skin cancers. Indeed, vitamin D has been shown to prevent prostate, colon, and breast cancers. Because of this, some doctors suggest ten to fifteen minutes of unprotected sun exposure several days a week to ensure that the body produces adequate amounts of vitamin D.

However, most dermatologists and skin cancer experts disagree with this. Even brief exposure to intense UV radiation can damage DNA and increase the risk of skin cancer. In addition, only a small amount of UV radiation is needed to make vitamin D. Even with a moderate-SPF sunscreen (SPF 15 or 30), enough UV radiation penetrates the skin for vitamin D production, according to an article in the *American Journal of Clinical Nutrition*. Also, the skin only makes a small amount of this vitamin at a time. Increasing the amount of UV radiation exposure does not lead to more vitamin D, only more DNA damage. Lastly, a variety of foods contain vitamin D, including salmon, tuna, beef, and eggs. Many foods have been fortified with vitamin D, including orange juice, milk, and other dairy products. People who have very limited sun exposure, who have dairy allergies, or who don't eat animal products, including fish, eggs, and dairy, should consult with a health care provider about possible vitamin D supplements.

Myths and Facts

I don't need to wear sunscreen if it is cloudy.

Fact: ➡ Depending on the moisture levels, some UV radiation can pass through clouds even when visible sunlight is blocked. In addition, UV radiation can bounce off the sides of dense clouds, actually increasing the amount of UV radiation reaching the surface. The SCF recommends wearing sunscreen daily when outdoors, even when it is cloudy.

Since I feel good after getting a tan, it must be good for me.

Fact: ➡ While a small amount of UV radiation helps promote vitamin D production, large amounts damage DNA and can lead to skin cancers. Some scientists believe that tanning can also lead to the production of endorphins, which are natural chemicals produced in our bodies that make us feel good. This "natural high" can be addictive and make some people tan excessively, a condition sometimes referred to as "tanorexia." Indeed, according to research published in the *Journal of the American Academy of Dermatology*, this addiction can be so strong that blocking this behavior can lead to withdrawal symptoms, such as nausea and jitteriness, in some individuals.

I don't have to worry about skin cancer until I'm older.

Fact: ➡ While it is true that most cases of skin cancer are among people older than sixty-five, people younger than twenty develop skin cancer as well. In fact, the rate of skin cancer in the younger population is increasing. According to the FDA, melanoma, the deadliest form of skin cancer, is linked to getting severe sunburns, especially at a young age.

four

HOW IS SKIN CANCER TREATED?

Skin cancers are often first noticed when a new or unusual lesion appears on the skin. Some people might ignore these changes, perhaps because they do not understand the potential dangers of skin cancer. But having any skin lesions evaluated by a health professional, especially at early stages, can help ensure the best possible outcomes. Health professionals can properly diagnose skin lesions to determine if they're cancerous. Then they educate and guide their patients in choosing the most effective treatment options.

Diagnosis

To determine which treatment is the best for each case, physicians first learn what type of skin cancer it is, how large the tumor is, and whether the cancer has spread.

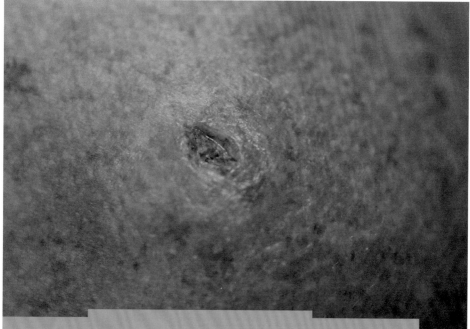

When physicians encounter suspicious skin lesions like this, they often perform a biopsy by cutting out a small section so that it may be examined more closely under a microscope.

Biopsies (in which a small area of the skin is removed and studied) allow health professionals to examine a suspicious area and find out if it is indeed cancerous. Using powerful microscopes, specialists can distinguish between normal, healthy cells and cancerous ones and estimate the size of the tumor. In cases of small cancers, the biopsy itself can cure the cancer if the whole tumor is removed.

If a physician is suspicious that a cancer has spread, a sentinel node biopsy is sometimes performed. When cancers metastasize, they often travel throughout the body via the lymphatic system, which helps remove waste and debris from tissues. Lymph nodes may filter and capture some of the cancerous cells. For this reason, a physician may remove several lymph nodes near the site of the cancer. Similar to a skin biopsy, cancer specialists examine the nodes for cancer cells, whose presence would suggests the tumor has metastasized to other organs. Occasionally, imaging such as X-rays, CT scans, or MRIs may be used to search for metastasis in other organs.

Using this information, a physician will stage the cancer using the American Joint Committee on Cancer's TMN system. "TMN" refers to (1) tumor size, (2) whether the cancer has metastasized, and (3) whether the cancer has spread to nearby lymph nodes. The cancer is ranked from Stage 0 (an extremely small cancer with no spread to lymph nodes or other organs) to Stage IV (a very large tumor that has invaded nearby organs, such as muscles and bones, and has spread to distant organs, such as the lungs or brain). Stage 0 and Stage I skin cancers are highly curable and carry an excellent prognosis, while Stage III and Stage IV cancers require aggressive therapy and have lower chances of being cured.

Therapies

The most effective treatment for a patient's skin cancer will depend on the type of cancer, the stage of cancer, its location, and the patient's overall health. Treatment options are not mutually exclusive, and doctors may use several different therapies at once, especially in high-stage cancers.

The stages of melanoma

Melanoma is a skin cancer of the pigment cells. The stages of the disease:

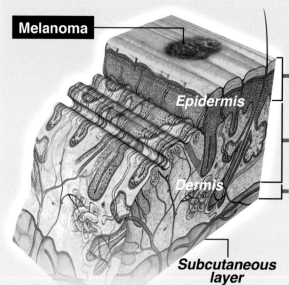

Melanoma

Epidermis

Dermis

Subcutaneous layer

STAGE I
Cancer in the outer layer of skin, the epidermis; tumor thickness less than 1/16 inch (1.5 mm)

STAGE II
Spreads to inner layer, the dermis; tumor thickness less than 1/6 inch (4 mm) thick

STAGE III
In tissue below skin **or** tumor more than 1/6 inch (4 mm) thick **or** cancer spread to lymph nodes, part of the immune system

STAGE IV
Spreads to major organs or to lymph nodes far from original tumor

Lymph nodes

Skin cancer types

There are several types of skin cancer. Melanoma is the least common but most fatal.

4% — Share of cases

96%

Deaths

21%

79%

■ **Melanoma**
☐ **Other skin cancers**

SOURCES: American Cancer Society, Current Medical Diagnosis and Treatment, Melanoma Patients Information Page Web site
Research/JUDY TREIBLE, Graphic/TODD LINDEMAN

© 2000 KRT

The prognosis of melanoma depends on its stage. Stage I cancers are highly curable. Unfortunately, Stage IV melanomas are difficult to treat and are associated with a high death rate.

Surgery

Surgical options are the most common treatment for skin cancers. Excising, or cutting out, the cancer will usually cure low-stage cancers, including melanomas. Cancer specialists will examine the removed tumor for the presence of margins. By observing layers of normal, cancer-free cells completely surrounding the tumor, the physician ensures that all cancerous cells were removed. Because cancer cells grow so quickly and aggressively, even a single cell left behind could cause trouble in the future. If the physician doesn't see a sufficient margin for the first excision, the area may have to be re-excised to ensure complete removal of the tumor.

On cosmetically important parts of the body, such as the face, the doctor's goal is to remove the tumor completely while leaving as much healthy skin behind as he or she safely can. Physicians often require a smaller margin of healthy cells when removing tumors from the face. One surgical technique, called Mohs surgery, involves removing the tumor one layer at a time and examining each layer under a microscope until only healthy cells are seen. While this technique can be time-consuming, it removes less skin and leaves smaller scars than traditional excisions.

For very superficial tumors, a doctor may perform cryosurgery, in which extremely cold liquid nitrogen is applied to freeze and kill cancer cells. Cryosurgery is often used for the treatment of precancerous actinic keratoses.

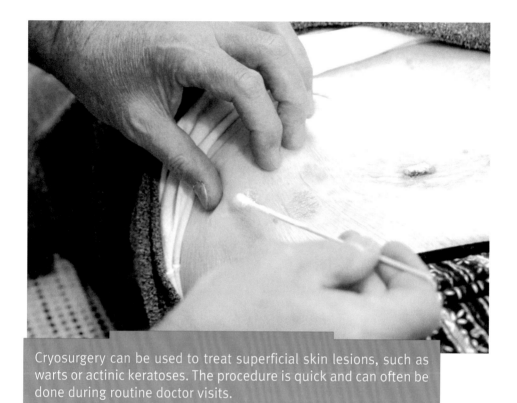

Cryosurgery can be used to treat superficial skin lesions, such as warts or actinic keratoses. The procedure is quick and can often be done during routine doctor visits.

Medications and Chemotherapy

Medications may be used to treat skin cancers. Often, these work by attacking cells that are growing rapidly. Imiquimod and 5-fluorouracil are two topical medications that may be applied directly to the tumor. They are often used for superficial BCCs. Other medications may be given by mouth or may be injected into veins.

Doctors often use chemotherapy for high-stage cancers, especially advanced melanomas. Because these drugs travel

Chemotherapy medications, such as cisplatin, work by targeting rapidly growing cells. They are effective in treating metastatic cancers, although they often have significant side effects.

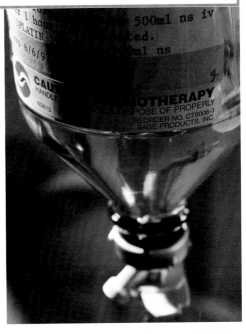

throughout the body, they can attack skin cancer cells that have metastasized to other organs. Chemotherapy is often given in cycles with rest periods to allow the body to recover. Some chemotherapy medications include dacarbazine (also called DTIC), cisplatin, and vinblastine. As scientists' understanding of skin cancer grows, so do the number of newer and more effective chemotherapies available.

The side effects of chemotherapy are unpleasant for many people, but they are usually temporary and go away after the treatments. The most common side effects are nausea, vomiting, diarrhea, and hair loss. Also, patients undergoing chemotherapy often experience unintentional weight loss. Fatigue is another common side effect: patients will often have anemia because the chemotherapy may prevent new red blood cells from developing. Likewise, there is an increased risk of infections as chemotherapy can cause decreased production of white blood cells, which fight infection. There is also an increased chance of bleeding and bruising due to decreased production of the platelets responsible for clotting blood. If chemotherapy causes hair loss, the patient's hair will begin to grow again when the chemotherapy is completed. The exact side effects of chemotherapy vary somewhat from drug to drug and from person to person.

Radiation Therapy

Another treatment option is radiation therapy. This treatment focuses high-energy radiation in a small area to kill cancerous cells. It is painless and usually takes only a few minutes. Radiation kills cancer cells by damaging their DNA. There is a risk that nearby healthy cells can become mutated and cancerous following treatment, however.

Radiation therapy is usually not used to treat tumors on the skin, although it is sometimes tried if a melanoma recurs in the original site after excision. More often, radiation therapy is used to treat metastases to other organs, such as the brain or bones. Side effects depend on what areas of the body are exposed to the radiation. Sometimes, there may be a sunburnlike effect on the skin. Other side effects include nausea, vomiting, fatigue, and hair loss. Like the side effects of chemotherapy, these are temporary.

Immunotherapy

A newer treatment that is getting a lot of attention is immunotherapy. This therapy involves boosting the immune system to recognize and attack tumors.

Immune cells use two chemicals called interferon alpha and interleukin-2 to communicate. When extra amounts of these

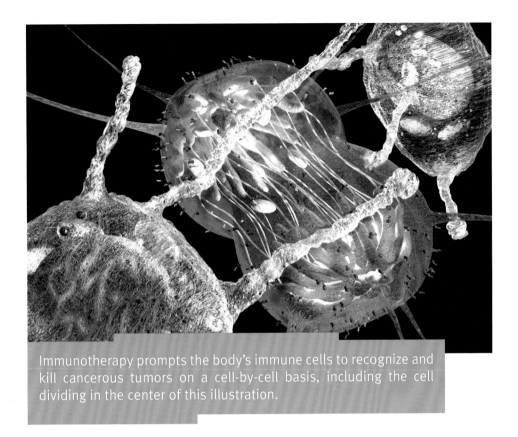

Immunotherapy prompts the body's immune cells to recognize and kill cancerous tumors on a cell-by-cell basis, including the cell dividing in the center of this illustration.

chemicals are given to cancer patients, they are sometimes effective in killing tumors. Immunotherapy has been effective in shrinking tumors in about 20 percent of patients with high-stage melanomas. Side effects include flulike symptoms, including fevers and aches.

Ipilimumab, a synthetic antibody, stimulates T cells into attacking cancer cells. In clinical trials, high-stage melanoma patients taking ipilimumab lived longer. It is now being studied in low-stage cancers. An uncommon, but dangerous, side effect of ipilimumab is that the immune system may become overstimulated and attack healthy cells as well. This effect can be fatal, but corticosteroids, which suppress the immune reaction, may be given to reverse it.

Complementary and Alternative Therapies

Besides the therapies discussed above, many cancer patients seek out complementary and alternative therapies. Complementary therapies are ones used in addition to standard medical therapy. For example, some patients may use acupuncture or receive massages to reduce stress. Or, patients may drink peppermint tea to help alleviate nausea from chemotherapy.

Alternative therapies are those that are performed instead of medical therapies. People who seek out alternative therapies may mistrust medical professionals, or they may have been given false hope and misinformation from individuals selling the therapy. Many alternative therapies have not been evaluated by the FDA, or if they have, they have been found ineffective.

Skin cancer is highly curable if found and treated early, but seeking alternative treatments first may lead to unnecessary delays. When considering alternative and complementary therapies, it is important to gather as much information as possible to make informed decisions. Medical professionals are an invaluable resource in answering any questions about skin cancer therapies.

Ten Great Questions to Ask a Doctor

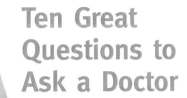

1 What type of skin cancer do I have?

2 What is my prognosis?

3 Are there other doctors I need to see?

4 What are the different treatment options for my cancer?

5 What are the risks and benefits of each?

6 What side effects should I expect from the treatment?

7 What should I do to prepare for the treatments?

What are the chances I will have a new skin tumor in the future?

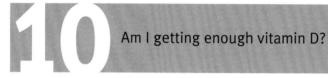 What strength of sunscreen would you recommend?

10 Am I getting enough vitamin D?

five

HOW WILL HAVING SKIN CANCER AFFECT MY LIFE?

In general, the chances of surviving skin cancer are very good when it is recognized and addressed early on. If initial treatments do not work, physicians can attempt more aggressive therapies. There are constantly new medications being developed, including potentially powerful ones that specifically target skin cancer cells with minimal side effects. Occasionally, however, some cancers become resistant to these treatments, and curing the patient becomes less likely, especially if the cancer has already spread to the lungs or brain.

Also, it is important to consider the benefits of performing more treatments compared to the side effects and the impact on the patient's quality of life. If a cure is not possible, treatments should aim to ease the symptoms. In palliative care,

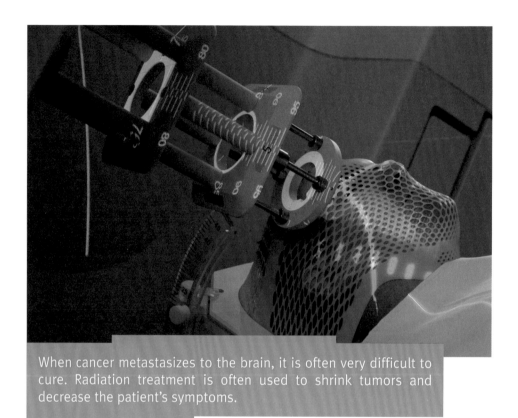

When cancer metastasizes to the brain, it is often very difficult to cure. Radiation treatment is often used to shrink tumors and decrease the patient's symptoms.

the goal is to help the patient feel as good as possible for as long as possible. This may include using some of the same therapies used to try to cure skin cancer, but with different goals. For example, radiation therapy may be used to shrink tumors and decrease pain.

Even for the many people who survive skin cancer, the worry about recurrence after an effective treatment can be extremely stressful. For example, half of BCC patients will have a new skin cancer within five years. Regular follow-up appointments with a health care provider are essential. Typically, these follow-ups are very frequent (every three to six months) after the initial treatment for the first several years. During these visits, the skin and lymph nodes are examined. Occasionally, imaging, such as X-rays or CT scans, may be necessary to confirm that there are no tumors growing in other organs. A skin cancer survivor should also be doing monthly self-examinations of the skin and lymph nodes. Any new symptoms that do not go away, including loss of appetite, nausea, aches, skin changes, or cough, should be brought to a health care provider's attention immediately.

Lifestyle Changes

Many people who learn of a cancer diagnosis take time to examine and evaluate their lives. This is particularly true for teenagers and young adults, who realize they are not as invulnerable as they may have believed. Many take this opportunity to develop healthy habits.

Exercise can help fight depression, anxiety, and fatigue, which are all common among those undergoing cancer treatment. It has been shown to lower the risk of some types of cancer, including colon, lung, and breast cancers. The ACS recommends at least thirty minutes of moderate physical activity five days a week. Exercising with a friend is an excellent way to stay motivated and have fun. Individuals should consult a health care provider before starting a new exercise program, especially during treatment.

Healthy eating is another lifestyle change that many cancer survivors embrace. Fruits and vegetables contain antioxidants and fiber, both of which have been shown to reduce the risk of many cancers. Eating more whole grains and less processed meats and sugars are also important parts of a cancer survivor's diet. Other significant cancer risk factors should be eliminated, including smoking and drinking alcohol. Reducing stress and finding time to relax are other key steps, as quality rest is critical for a healthy body.

These healthy lifestyle changes can reduce a person's risk for many cancers. Unfortunately, there is no evidence that these lifestyle changes will reduce the risk of a recurrence in a person with skin cancer. Most research focuses on the importance of primary prevention: avoiding UV radiation from the sun and tanning booths. Some cancer survivors use their experiences to educate others about the causes of skin cancer. For example, Samantha Hessel developed a melanoma on her elbow at the age of nineteen because of her frequent visits to tanning beds. Now she is an advocate for the Melanoma Research Foundation (MRF) and warns others about the dangers of indoor tanning.

Emotional Health

Even with an excellent prognosis, living with cancer can be very scary. Sometimes, learning about a cancer diagnosis can trigger an episode of depression. Symptoms of depression include significant changes in appetite (eating much more or much less than normal), changes in sleep (either sleeping much more than usual or getting very little sleep), loss of energy, loss of interest in activities that one used to enjoy, and an inability to concentrate. While some degree of depression is understandable after learning about a cancer diagnosis, people with severe depression often have a difficult time getting through the day,

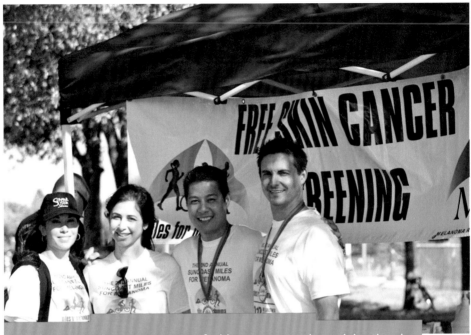

Working to raise awareness of skin cancer and participating in fund-raising events are powerful ways people can help fight the most common cancer.

performing their jobs, schoolwork, family responsibilities, or even caring for themselves appropriately. Talking to a health care provider or a therapist can help a cancer patient overcome depression. There are therapists who are specifically trained in counseling individuals with cancer, as well as helping family members of cancer patients. Thoughts about hurting oneself are very serious symptoms of depression, and they should be brought to a health care provider's attention immediately.

While health professionals are very knowledgeable about the science of skin cancer, few of them have actually been treated for it themselves. Health care providers can sometimes forget how overwhelming and intimidating some of the treatments may sound, especially to a teenager or young adult. Cancer patients should always feel encouraged to ask questions and express their fears to health professionals. It is also important to have the emotional support of family and friends. Talking to a close friend or family member often gives cancer patients extra strength and courage during difficult times.

With over two million patients diagnosed yearly, according to the American Academy of Dermatology, skin cancer is the most common cancer. There are many survivors who are willing to share their experiences, both to educate others and to lend emotional support. Talking to cancer survivors about their personal experiences can help lower anxiety and build courage. Some may have useful advice, such as how to deal with the side effects of some therapies. Health care providers who specialize in treating skin cancers often have contact information for local communities of skin cancer survivors. The ACS provides information on finding local groups on its Web site, http://www.cancer.org. While being diagnosed with skin cancer may be scary, it should never be lonely.

Skin cancers are a significant worry for teenagers and young adults. But education can be an important defense. Understanding and minimizing risk factors for skin cancer, especially UV radiation exposure, can prevent future occurrences of skin cancer. Being aware of changes on one's skin, and having a health professional evaluate any suspicious lesions early, increases the likelihood of a successful outcome. Armed with knowledge and fortified with a healthy lifestyle, a skin cancer survivor can expect a long and fulfilling life.

anemia A condition in which the blood has fewer oxygen-carrying red blood cells than normal, which often results in a person feeling weak and tired.

antioxidant A molecule that protects cells from the damaging effects of ionizing radiation and free radicals (highly reactive atoms that can damage cells, proteins, and DNA by altering their chemical structure).

benign Not cancerous; presenting no danger to health or well-being.

biopsy The removal and examination of a small sample of tissue from the body in order to check for disease.

carcinogen A substance that has been shown to cause DNA damage and increase the risk of developing cancer.

CT scan Computed tomography scan; high-resolution X-rays that enable health professionals to get a highly detailed, three-dimensional view of the inside of a patient's body. Also may be referred to as a CAT scan.

DNA Deoxyribonucleic acid; the genetic information in each cell that contains the blueprints for how each cell should function.

gene A portion of DNA that contains information on one specific trait, such as eye color, how to make a certain protein, or how fast a cell should grow.

lesion An abnormal, injured, or diseased spot or area on or in the body.

lymph node A small, bean-shaped organ that helps filter fluids in the body and aids in fighting infections.

malignant Cancerous, with the potential to invade other parts of the body and possibly cause death.

margin Layers of healthy noncancerous cells surrounding a tumor in a biopsy specimen.

metabolism The chemical processes occurring within a living cell or organism that are necessary to sustain life.

metastasize To spread from the original site of cancerous cells to another part of the body.

mortality The likelihood that a person with a disease will die from that disease within a certain time period.

MRI Magnetic resonance imaging; the use of magnetic waves to obtain highly detailed pictures of internal organs.

mutation A change in the DNA of a gene.

platelet A fragment of specialized blood cells that aid in blood clotting.

prognosis The outcome of a disease; the likelihood that a cancer will be successfully treated.

recurrence The return or reappearance of symptoms of a disease.

risk factor An element, such as a behavior, which has been shown to increase the likelihood of developing a disease.

stage A classification of a malignant tumor based on its size and how much it has spread.

superficial Situated on or near the surface.

American Academy of Dermatology (AAD)
930 East Woodfield Road
Schaumburg, IL 60173
(888) 462-DERM [3376]
Web site: http://www.aad.org
  The AAD provides facts and recommendations on keeping
  skin healthy and beautiful, including tips for preventing skin
  cancer. Directories on the organization's Web site will help you
  locate nearby dermatologists and free skin cancer screenings.

American Cancer Society (ACS)
250 Williams Street NW
Atlanta, GA 30303
(800) 227-2345
Web site: http://www.cancer.org
  The ACS has a wealth of information about the causes
  and treatments of many cancers, including new treatments currently undergoing clinical trials. It also offers
  information about contacting local cancer support groups.

Canadian Cancer Society
55 St. Clair Avenue West, Suite 300
Toronto, ON M4V 2Y7
Canada
(416) 961-7223

Web site: http://www.cancer.ca
  The Canadian Cancer Society is a community-based program
  whose goal is the support and enrichment of the lives of
  people with cancer.

Canadian Dermatology Association
1385 Bank Street, Suite 425
Ottawa, ON K1H 8N4
Canada
(800) 267-3376
Web site: http://www.dermatology.ca
  The Canadian Dermatology Association promotes research
  on skin health and provides public information on sun exposure and skin care.

Melanoma Research Foundation
1411 K Street NW, Suite 500
Washington, DC 20005
(800) 673-1290
Web site: http://www.melanoma.org
  The Melanoma Research Foundation is committed to educat-
  ing physicians and the public about the causes and
  consequences of melanoma.

National Cancer Institute
6116 Executive Boulevard, Suite 300
Bethesda, MD 20892
(800) 4-CANCER [422-6237]
Web site: http://www.cancer.gov

The National Cancer Institute funds and supports research into the prevention and treatment of all cancer types, and it distributes new cancer information to the public.

Skin Cancer Foundation (SCF)

149 Madison Avenue, Suite 901

New York, NY 10016

(212) 725-5176

Web site: http://www.skincancer.org
  The SCF is an international organization dedicated to education about and prevention of skin cancers.

Web Sites

Due to the changing nature of Internet links, Rosen Publishing has developed an online list of Web sites related to the subject of this book. This site is updated regularly. Please use this link to access the list:

http://www.rosenlinks.com/faq/scan

American Cancer Society. *Melanoma Skin Cancer: What You Need to Know—Now* (Quick Facts). Atlanta, GA: American Cancer Society/Health Promotions, 2012.

Brezina, Corona. *Frequently Asked Questions About Tanning and Skin Care* (FAQ: Teen Life). New York, NY: Rosen Publishing, 2010.

Buckmaster, Marjorie L. *Skin Cancer* (Health Alert). New York, NY: Marshall Cavendish Benchmark, 2008.

Fredericks, Carrie, ed. *Skin Cancer* (Perspectives on Diseases and Disorders). Farmington Hills, MI: Greenhaven Press, 2010.

Goldsmith, Connie. *Skin Cancer* (USA TODAY Health Reports). Minneapolis, MN: Twenty-First Century Books, 2011.

Jaworski, Sabina K., and Robert Chehoski. *Skin Care* (Girls' Health). New York, NY: Rosen Central, 2012.

Juettner, Bonnie. *Skin Cancer* (Diseases and Disorders). Detroit, MI: Lucent Books, 2008.

Mukherjee, Siddhartha. *The Emperor of All Maladies: A Biography of Cancer.* New York, NY: Scribner, 2010.

So, Po-Lin. *Skin Cancer* (Biology of Cancer). New York, NY: Chelsea House, 2008.

Wang, Steven Q. *Beating Melanoma: A Five-Step Survival Guide.* Baltimore, MD: Johns Hopkins University Press, 2009.

About the Author

John M. Shea has earned both a medical degree and a Ph.D. in biochemistry and molecular biology from the Medical University of South Carolina. He has always had a fascination with medicine and the science of how our bodies work. Recently, he has turned his attention to writing for children and young adults in the hope of sharing his enthusiasm for the wonders of human biology. When he is not writing health and science books, he can usually be found loudly cheering for the Buffalo Sabres.

Photo Credits

Cover © iStockphoto.com/Anagramm; p. 6 udaix/Shutterstock.com; p. 8 Peter Dazeley/Photographer's Choice/Getty Images; p. 9 individual photos courtesy Skin Cancer Foundation; p. 12 Convit/Shutterstock.com; p. 16 Steve Gschmeissner/Science Photo Library/Getty Images; p. 19 Dorling Kindersley/Getty Images; p. 21 Brand X Pictures/Getty Images; pp. 25, 40 Joe Raedle/Getty Images; p. 28 © iStockphoto.com/Johnnyhetfield; p. 31 © iStockphoto.com/Graça Victoria; p. 34 ©iStockphoto.com/Sieto Verver; p. 42 Lindeman/KRT/Newscom; p. 44 Antonia Reeve/Photo Researchers, Inc.; p. 45 Mark Harmel/Stone/Getty Images; p. 47 © XVIVO LLC/Phototake; p. 52 Mark Kostich/Vetta/Getty Images; p. 55 Courtesy Melanoma Research Foundation.

Designer: Evelyn Horovicz; Editor: Andrea Sclarow Paskoff; Photo Researcher: Marty Levick